CIRRHOSIS DIET COOKBOOK FOR NEWLY DIAGNOSED

The Nutritional Guide with Delicious Recipes to Detoxify and Revitalize your Liver and Live Healthy

TABLE OF CONTENT

INTRODUCTION

This is a carefully curated nutritious diet cookbook with cornerstones of a complete approach to healthiness that is necessary for people with cirrhosis. I recognize the challenges that cirrhosis presents and aim to empower you with the knowledge and tools needed to make informed choices.

Cirrhosis is a condition in which the liver experiences increasing scarring, in this book, I will take you on a journey to understand cirrhosis covering everything from its causes and origins to the complex dance it does inside the body.

In addition, I will discuss the complex connection between cirrhosis and nutrition and demonstrate the significant benefits of a balanced diet for both cirrhosis management and general well-being.

I'll break down the complexity of cirrhosis in the pages that follow, offering details on its different manifestations, symptoms, and possible side effects. You will learn the value of early detection, professional diagnosis, and a comprehensive understanding of the illness to enable you to make well-informed decisions on your path to improved health.

Crucially, this book is not just a guide to cirrhosis; it's a companion on your path to wellness. Whether you're seeking to manage cirrhosis or are proactively adopting a liver-friendly lifestyle, this cookbook is your roadmap to a healthier, more vibrant you.

So, let's embark on this transformative journey together, embracing the power of food as a source of healing and strength.

Your kitchen is about to become a haven of health, and your plate, a canvas for nourishment. Here's to a vibrant, flavorful, and fulfilling life.

CHAPTER ONE

UNDERSTANDING LIVER CIRRHOSIS

How Cirrhosis Affect the Liver

Liver cirrhosis is a late-stage liver condition in which scar tissue has progressively replaced healthy liver tissue.

This is the outcome of chronic, long-term hepatitis. There are numerous causes of hepatitis, which is an inflammation of the liver. When inflammation persists, your liver tries to heal itself by creating scars. However, an excess of scar tissue impairs liver function. Prolonged liver failure is the final stage.

Cirrhosis is a progressive condition that worsens as more and more scar tissue develops.

In the beginning, your body adjusts to compensate for your reduced liver function, and you might not notice it too much. This is known as compensated cirrhosis. Eventually, though, as your liver function declines further, you will begin to experience noticeable symptoms. This is known as decompensated cirrhosis.

Scarring in your liver blocks the flow of blood and oxygen through your liver tissues. This slows your liver's ability to process your blood, metabolize nutrients and filter out toxins. Cirrhosis reduces your liver's ability to produce bile and essential blood proteins. Scar tissue can also compress blood vessels running through your liver, including the important portal vein system, leading to a condition called portal hypertension.

The development of cirrhosis is attributed to a number of causes and risk factors. For the purposes of prevention, early identification, and efficient management, is essential! The following are some typical cirrhosis causes and risk factors;

Chronic Alcohol Consumption

Persistently engaging in excessive and prolonged alcohol consumption stands as a primary and predominant contributor to the onset of cirrhosis.

Chronic alcohol consumption has a deleterious effect on the liver due to a number of disease processes. At first, inflammation takes hold and fosters an environment that is favorable to liver damage.

Long-term heavy alcohol consumption can also cause fatty liver, which is defined by the buildup of fat inside liver cells. This first phase, called alcoholic fatty liver disease, is a prelude to more serious disorders that culminate in the formation of cirrhosis.

The final stage of chronic liver damage brought on by heavy and persistent alcohol use is known as alcohol-induced cirrhosis. The normal architecture of the liver is disrupted by the scarring associated with cirrhosis, hence impairing its critical activities.

This complex chain reaction highlights the seriousness of the repercussions linked to long-term alcohol misuse.

It important you know this in order to be aware of how much alcohol you should consume in order to reduce your chances of developing cirrhosis and other liver diseases.

Chronic Viral Hepatitis

Sustained infections with either the hepatitis B or C viruses constitute a significant risk factor for the development of chronic viral hepatitis.

This prolonged inflammatory state, if left unchecked, can set the stage for the gradual progression towards cirrhosis.

A long-lasting and dynamic interplay between the immune system and the viral agents, hepatitis B or C, is represented by chronic viral hepatitis.

These viruses' continuous attack on the liver tissues causes and maintains inflammation, which fosters the environment that leads to progressive liver damage.

This ongoing inflammatory reaction has the potential to cause fibrous tissue to progressively replace healthy liver tissue over time, ultimately leading to the development of cirrhosis.

Non-alcoholic Fatty Liver Disease (NAFLD)

Non-alcoholic Fatty Liver Disease (NAFLD) emerges as a distinct medical condition typified by the progressive accumulation of excess fat within the liver. This aberrant lipid deposition, if left unaddressed, can manifest in its more advanced and severe manifestation known as non-alcoholic steatohepatitis (NASH).

It is within the realm of NASH that the risks escalate, potentially paving the way for the development of cirrhosis, an advanced stage characterized by irreversible scarring of the liver tissue.

The aetiology of non-alcoholic fatty liver disease (NAFLD) is closely associated with many metabolic variables, wherein obesity and metabolic syndrome are prominent risk factors.

The complex interaction between lifestyle choices and the metabolic processes of the liver is significantly upset, which results in the abnormal build-up of fat in the liver cells.

The continuous evolution of non-alcoholic fatty liver disease (NAFLD) is initiated by this metabolic imbalance, which is further exacerbated by obesity and metabolic syndrome. As NAFLD advances to its more severe counterpart, NASH, the risk of cirrhosis becomes an imminent concern.

Recognizing the role of obesity and metabolic syndrome as common risk factors further emphasizes the need for a holistic approach to liver health that addresses underlying metabolic imbalances and promotes overall well-being.

Genetic Disorders

Genetic disorders, encompassing a spectrum of hereditary conditions, play a pivotal role in the predisposition towards cirrhosis.

Among these hereditary conditions, notable examples include hemochromatosis, a genetic disorder marked by the excessive accumulation of iron within the liver, and Wilson's disease, a condition characterized by abnormal copper metabolism.

Additionally, alpha-1 antitrypsin deficiency, another genetic anomaly, stands as a contributing factor to the progression of cirrhosis. Understanding the hereditary roots of these conditions highlights the significance of a customized and all-encompassing strategy for liver health.

Long-Term Exposure to Toxins and Drugs

The liver, being a central organ in detoxification and metabolism, is uniquely susceptible to the impact of prolonged exposure to various substances.

Certain environmental toxins, when encountered persistently, can overwhelm the liver's detoxification capabilities, triggering a cascade of adverse effects that may ultimately lead to tissue scarring characteristic of cirrhosis.

Similarly, the utilization of drugs that undergo extensive processing by the liver can exert a cumulative toll on its functionality, potentially culminating in liver damage and the progression towards cirrhosis.

This complex interaction between prolonged exposure to medications and toxins and the liver's vulnerability emphasizes how important you need to be vigilant and aware of the potential risks.

Some people who work in settings where exposure to toxins is high or who use medications that the liver metabolizes ought to be aware of the possible effects on liver health.

This knowledge serves as the basis for taking preventative action, requesting routine medical monitoring, and making educated decisions to protect the liver from the harmful consequences of extended exposure to chemicals and medications.

Cystic Fibrosis

If you are the type that is grappling with cystic fibrosis, a hereditary and chronic respiratory condition, there exists a potential vulnerability that you develop cirrhosis.

This susceptibility arises from the unique characteristic of cystic fibrosis, wherein thick and viscous mucus accumulates within various organs, including the liver. Although cystic fibrosis is well known for its effects on the respiratory system, it also affects other important organs, which has a wider range of consequences. One such organ that must deal with the unusually thick mucus generated. This mucus, which is well known for blocking different body pathways, can disrupt the normal flow of bile through the liver's network of ducts.

Symptoms and Diagnosis

Your ability to identify cirrhosis symptoms increases as your liver function deteriorates.

For instance, there may be indications that bile is overflowing into areas it shouldn't be and isn't going where it should be. Some of the symptoms are:

Nausea and Loss of Appetite

Although they may not appear like symptoms, nausea and decreased appetite may be more serious indicators of cirrhosis, a disorder in which the liver tissue gradually scars.

These seemingly benign symptoms turn become important markers, providing subtle clues about the complex alterations taking place in the liver and the more general physiological effects that can materialize in the future.

When cirrhosis is present, nausea is one of the symptoms that may be related to a number of conditions, such as liver damage, gastrointestinal issues, or consequences like ascites, which is an abnormal build-up of fluid in the abdominal cavity.

One of the main symptoms of cirrhosis is impaired liver function, which can cause disturbances in the digestive system and make one feel queasy.

Recognizing nausea and appetite loss as possible cirrhosis symptoms calls for a comprehensive approach to patient management.

In order to identify the underlying causes of these symptoms and develop customized therapies, regular medical monitoring, thorough diagnostics, and patient-provider communication are essential.

Feeling Generally Unwell

Malaise, which is a generalized feeling of being poorly, is one of the notable symptoms that may indicate cirrhosis underneath. This subtle discomfort goes beyond simple weariness or exhaustion to encompass a more comprehensive and systemic expression of the alterations taking place in the liver, which is gradually scarring.

There are several different causes of malaise in cirrhosis. The widespread sense of being unwell is the result of a systemic imbalance that is exacerbated by these interruptions.

Additionally, cirrhosis-related problems like portal hypertension or the onset of ascites can exacerbate the feeling of being unwell.

The body's entire equilibrium can be significantly impacted by the altered circulation and fluid imbalances linked to these issues, which can intensify the sensation of being unwell overall.

Finding the root causes of malaise requires routine medical evaluations, such as liver function testing and diagnostic imaging.

Upper abdominal pain (especially on the right)

Upper abdomen pain, especially on the right side, is a notable symptom that can indicate the beginning or development of cirrhosis. This discomfort is localized in the upper right quadrant of the abdomen, which is physically where the liver is placed.

It is frequently described as a dull, continuous ache. Investigating the complex dynamics of liver function and the effects of cirrhosis on the surrounding structures is necessary to comprehend this discomfort as a symptom.

It is crucial to recognize that the nature and intensity of upper abdominal pain can vary. You may experience a dull ache, while others may perceive a sharper, more acute pain.

Monitoring the onset and progression of this pain is essential, as it can serve as an important indicator of the evolving state of liver health. Understanding your upper abdominal pain is a symptom of cirrhosis prompts a proactive approach to healthcare.

Regular medical assessments, imaging studies, and consultations with healthcare providers are vital components in elucidating the underlying causes of this pain and devising tailored strategies for cirrhosis management.

Visible blood vessels that look like spiders

Spider angiomas, which are visible blood vessels that resemble spiders, are a unique and noticeable symptom that may indicate underlying cirrhosis.

Scientifically known as telangiectasias, these spider-like structures appear as tiny, reddish lesions with radiating blood vessels and a central arteriole that mimic the structure of a spider's web.

Deciphering the complex vascular and hemodynamic changes that take place in the liver is necessary to comprehend the existence of spider angiomas in the setting of cirrhosis.

Spider angiomas are particularly linked to the hemodynamic shifts associated with cirrhosis, specifically the changes in blood flow and pressure within the liver.

As cirrhosis progresses and scarring disrupts the normal architecture of the liver, blood flow is rerouted, leading to the formation of collateral vessels.

Spider angiomas, being a visible expression of these vascular changes, are a consequence of the increased pressure within the circulatory system, particularly in the portal vein.

The identification of spider angiomas as a sign of cirrhosis highlights the significance of an all-encompassing approach to patient care.

It becomes essential to do routine medical examinations, such as liver function tests and diagnostic imaging, in order to determine the underlying reasons of these vascular alterations.

These outward signs can also act as visual cues, encouraging people and medical professionals to learn more about the subtleties of liver health and develop specialized cirrhosis management plans.

Diagnosis and Tests

Blood tests

A panel of liver function tests can show signs of liver disease and liver failure.

These measure liver products like liver enzymes, proteins and bilirubin levels in your blood. Blood tests may also indicate specific diseases or known side effects, like reduced blood clotting.

Imaging tests

Imaging tests like an abdominal ultrasound, CT scan or MRI can show the size, shape and texture of your liver. A special type of imaging test called elastography uses ultrasound or MRI technology to measure the level of stiffness or fibrosis in your liver.

Liver biopsy

A liver biopsy is a minor procedure to take a small tissue sample from your liver to test in a lab. A healthcare provider can usually take the sample through a hollow needle.

While not always necessary, a liver biopsy can confirm cirrhosis and may help determine the cause.

CHAPTER TWO

A CIRRHOSIS-FRIENDLY PANTRY

Creating a pantry that is conducive to cirrhosis is an essential first step toward converting dietary guidelines into doable, routine behaviors.

Stocking Your Kitchen with Essentials

Fresh Produce

Prioritize a vibrant array of fresh fruits and vegetables, rich in vitamins and antioxidants. Opt for easy-to-digest options such as leafy greens, berries, and citrus fruits. These form the cornerstone of a nutrient-dense, cirrhosis-friendly diet.

Lean Proteins

Choose lean protein sources to reduce the strain on the liver.

Include skinless poultry, fish, legumes, and tofu. These protein options provide essential amino acids without the excessive workload associated with processing fatty meats.

Healthy Fats

Integrate healthy fats like avocados, olive oil, and nuts. These sources of monounsaturated fats provide essential nutrients without overwhelming the liver, supporting overall cardiovascular and metabolic health.

Low-Sodium Options

Mindful sodium intake is crucial for cirrhosis management. Opt for low-sodium varieties of canned goods, broths, and condiments. Fresh herbs, spices, and lemon can be flavorful alternatives for seasoning.

Dairy Alternatives

Consider lactose-free or plant-based milk alternatives to accommodate potential lactose intolerance that may arise with cirrhosis. These alternatives maintain the nutritional value without the digestive strain.

List of cirrhosis-friendly Foods items

- Fruits and vegetables (including a green leafy variety)
- Eggs, egg whites
- Cooked fish, particularly salmon, tuna, and mackerel that contain high omega3 fatty acids
- Skinless chicken or turkey
- Plenty of vegetable protein like beans and legumes such as chickpeas, black beans, soybeans, kidney beans
- Low-fat milk and yogurt

- Low-fat or fat-free cheese made with skim milk such as mozzarella cheese
- Unsalted nuts and seeds or nut butter
- Seeds such as quinoa, flaxseed, pumpkin seeds are excellent sources of protein
- Whole grains, that are a great source of fiber, include barley, brown rice, millet, and oatmeal
- Whole wheat bread, pasta, and cereals without added sugar.
- Tofu
- Margarine
- Olive oil, canola oil, and safflower oil contain unsaturated fats
- Fresh herbs (example - milk thistle)
- Garlic, ginger
- Coconut water

Setting up a kitchen that is supportive of preparing meals that are cirrhosis-friendly requires having the appropriate equipment. These appliances help to preserve the nutritious value of your food while also making cooking easier. Some of the kitchen tools that are needed are:

Blender

Invest in a high-quality blender or food processor to create smoothies, soups, and purees. These appliances facilitate the preparation of easily digestible and nutrient-rich meals, ensuring a diverse range of textures for those with specific dietary needs.

Steamer

A steamer is an invaluable tool for gently cooking vegetables, fish, and poultry.

This cooking method retains the nutritional content of foods while making them easier on the digestive system, a crucial consideration for individuals managing cirrhosis.

Sharp Knives

Sharp knives are essential for efficient and safe food preparation. Well-maintained knives make chopping fruits, vegetables, and proteins more manageable, allowing for precise cuts and reducing the risk of accidents.

Non-Stick Cookware

Opt for non-stick cookware to minimize the need for added fats during cooking. Non-stick pans are ideal for preparing cirrhosis-friendly meals without excessive oil, promoting healthier cooking methods.

Herb and Spice Grinder

Enhance the flavor of your meals with fresh herbs and spices. Invest in a grinder to create your spice blends, avoiding pre-packaged mixes that may contain hidden sodium or additives.

Measuring Tools

Accurate measurements are crucial for maintaining portion control and adhering to dietary guidelines. Use measuring cups and spoons to ensure precision in ingredient quantities, supporting a balanced and mindful approach to nutrition.

Food Scale

A food scale provides an additional layer of accuracy, especially when monitoring portion sizes of proteins, grains, and other ingredients.

This tool aids in maintaining a balanced and controlled intake, promoting overall dietary adherence.

Slow Cooker or Crockpot

These appliances are excellent for preparing cirrhosis-friendly meals with minimal effort. Slow cooking allows flavors to meld, creating delicious and easily digestible dishes without the need for constant supervision.

Cutting Boards and Mats

Use separate cutting boards and mats for different food groups to prevent cross-contamination. Color-coded boards for vegetables, proteins, and fruits ensure a hygienic and organized meal preparation process.

CHAPTER THREE

DIETING FOR CIRRHOSIS DIET

As you begin the process of controlling your cirrhosis, I understand how crucial it is to understand the basic ideas of a diet that is specifically designed to promote liver health.

Balancing Macronutrients in Cirrhosis Diet Fundamentals

Achieving a balanced macronutrient composition is essential to creating a diet that is helpful for people with cirrhosis. For those coping with cirrhosis, these macronutrients carbohydrates, proteins, and fats are essential for maintaining liver health, controlling symptoms, and enhancing general wellbeing.

Carbohydrates

Carbohydrates stand as a paramount source of energy, a fundamental necessity for sustaining day-to-day activities and overall well-being. In the context of cirrhosis, where metabolic functions may be compromised, the strategic incorporation of carbohydrates into the diet takes on heightened importance.

A judicious and balanced intake of complex carbohydrates, encompassing whole grains, fruits, and vegetables, becomes indispensable in maintaining a consistent and sustainable energy supply without imposing undue stress on the liver through the ingestion of excessive sugars.

Developing a strategic approach to carbohydrate consumption means intentionally prioritizing complex carbs over their refined counterparts. The main component of this strategy is choosing nutrient-dense foods including whole grains, legumes, and foods high in fiber.

In addition to providing energy, these options support digestive health by offering vital dietary fiber.

Incorporating these complex carbs also promotes a steady and balanced metabolic environment by reducing the likelihood of sudden spikes in blood sugar.

Proteins

Proteins are essential components required for the complex processes of tissue upkeep and repair in the human body.

A careful and nuanced strategy is necessary to meet the body's protein needs without unduly taxing the liver's complex tasks in the setting of cirrhosis, where the liver's ability to process proteins may be impaired.

Understanding how important proteins are to maintaining general health, especially when dealing with the difficulties that come with cirrhosis, emphasizes the necessity of a careful and well-rounded protein plan.

Creating a protein intake plan that works requires carefully choosing lean protein sources that supply the necessary amino acids without taxing the liver. The best options include fish, chicken, lentils, and tofu; each provides a range of nutrients essential for tissue integrity.

The key to this approach is consuming moderate amounts of protein throughout the day, spread out over several meals.

This methodical technique supports a steady and balanced supply of amino acids while also being in harmony with the body's natural cycle of nutrition usage. Furthermore, adding plant-based proteins becomes a strategic consideration as well, providing a source of protein that requires less liver metabolism.

Fat

Healthy fats have a function that goes beyond their caloric content. They play a crucial part in aiding in the absorption of nutrients and enhancing the body's overall metabolic process.

A conscious focus on the kind and makeup of fats becomes critical in the complex terrain of cirrhosis, where the liver's functions may be impaired. Knowing how important fats are to health, especially when it comes to cirrhosis, emphasizes how important it is to design a diet that puts the health of the liver and the cardiovascular system first.

Developing a successful fat-intake plan requires concentrating on unsaturated fats, which are known to have a positive effect on the heart and to have a negligible influence on liver function. The best options in this category include nutrient-dense foods like avocados, almonds, and olive oil, all of which provide important fatty acids without overtaxing the liver's biochemical functions.

Coconut Chocolate Avocado Pudding

Total Time: 25 minutes

Serves:2

Ingredients

- 1 ripe avocado
- ¼ cup unsweetened cocoa powder
- 1 tsp vanilla
- 3 tbsp honey
- ¼ cup coconut milk
- Sweetened, shredded coconut for garnish

Directions

- Add avocado, cocoa, vanilla, honey and coconut milk to a mixing bowl.avocado
- Blend with an electric mixer until well blended and creamy. When ready, it should have very few lumps.avocado pudding

- Chill for 15 minutes, then serve in a dessert bowl and top with shredded coconut.coconut avocado pudding

Crab Omelet with Avocado and Herbs

Crab Omelet with Avocado and Herbs

Total Time: 15 minutes

Serves: 1

Ingredients

- 3 eggs
- 1 tsp minced parsley, plus extra for garnish
- 1 tsp minced chives, plus extra for garnish
- ½ tsp sea or kosher salt
- ½ tsp cracked black pepper
- 1 tbsp butter
- ½ oz shredded parmesan, about 2 tbsp
- 2 oz lump crab meat, about ½ cup
- 1 green onion, thinly sliced
- ½ avocado, sliced

- 1 tbsp sour cream

Directions

- Crack the eggs into a small bowl. Add the chives, parsley, salt, and pepper to the eggs, then whisk with a fork until frothy.
- Heat a 10″ non-stick skillet over medium heat. Add the butter, and swirl until it melts then foams. Once the foam subsides, pour the whisked eggs into the pan. Swirl the pan to cover the bottom with an even layer of eggs.
- Saute the eggs over medium heat until the edges are firm and the center is just barely cooked through, 3-4 minutes. Deflate any large bubbles with the tines of a fork.

- Sprinkle half the parmesan cheese over one half of the omelet. Top the cheese with the lump crab meat, then sprinkle with green onions. Layer the avocado over the green onions, then top with the remaining parmesan cheese.

- Using a spatula, fold the empty half of the eggs over to form a half circle. Remove from heat, and transfer to a plate. Sprinkle with additional fresh herbs to taste, and garnish with a dollop of sour cream. Serve immediately.

Spicy Omelet With Mushrooms

Total Time: 10 minutes

Serves: 2

Ingredients

- 4 eggs large
- 4 tablespoon olive oil
- 1 cup mushrooms
- 1 cup red bell pepper chopped
- 1 jalapeno pepper
- pinch salt
- pinch black pepper
- pinch cayenne pepper optional
- pinch garlic powder

Directions

- Chop the red bell pepper and jalapeno peppers. Wash and pat the mushrooms dry with a paper towel.
- Add a little oil to a pan or small skillet.

- Mix the spices in a small bowl. Add a pinch of salt and pepper and saute mushrooms and peppers for about 5 minutes, till soft.
- When done, take out the veggies and set them aside.
- Add some more olive oil to the frying pan. Break the eggs in a small bowl, add a pinch of the mixed spices, and whisk with a wire whisk.
- Pour the beaten eggs into the pan and let them cook on medium-high heat.
- Once the edges of the omelet begin to cook, tilt the pan slightly, so the uncooked egg runs to the edge of the skillet.
- Every few seconds, tilt the pan slightly so the egg keeps flowing to the edge.

- Cover the pan for about 30 seconds on medium heat if the top is not yet cooked through.
- Add the topping to half of the omelet.
- Fold the other half of the egg over the veggies using a rubber spatula. Turn off the heat and leave the pan covered for about a minute.
- Slide omelet onto your serving plate, and breakfast is ready!

Banana Oatmeal

Total Time: 15 minutes

Serves: 2

Ingredients

- 1 cup rolled oats
- 1 cup almond milk (or any type of milk)
- 1 cup water
- 1 spotty ripe banana, mashed

- 1 tbsp maple syrup (optional)
- 1 tsp vanilla extract
- 1 tsp cinnamon
- 1/8 tsp salt
- Toppings of choice (fresh fruit, nut butter, nuts, seeds, etc.)

Directions

- Combine all ingredients in a small pot.
- Transfer the pot to a stovetop and cook over medium-high heat. Frequently stir the oatmeal so it does not stick to the bottom of the pot. Cook until thick and creamy, about 7-8 minutes. The longer you cook, the thicker and creamier it will become.
- Transfer oatmeal to bowl(s). Add your favorite toppings, like fresh fruit, nut butter, granola, nuts, seeds, and more. Enjoy!

Total Time: 15 minutes

Serves: 1

Ingredients

- 1 small onion, sliced
- 6-8 medium mushrooms, sliced
- 150 g grassfed ground beef
- Salt and pepper to taste
- ½ tsp smoked paprika
- 2 eggs, lightly beaten
- 1 small avocado, diced
- 10-12 pitted black olives, sliced

Directions

- In a heavy skillet set over medium high heat melt a little bit of coconut oil. When oil is nice and hot, add onions, mushrooms, salt and pepper and cook until the veggies are

- fragrant and softened, about 2-3 minutes.
- Add ground beef and smoked paprika and continue cooking until the beef is no longer pink. Remove that to a plate.
- Add eggs to the skillet and scramble them to your liking.
- Return beef to the pan, add avocado and sliced olives.
- Continue cooking just to slightly warm up the avocados and olives, about 45 seconds to a minute.
- Transfer to a pretty bowl, garnish with parsley if desired, sit yourself down and enjoy!

Buckwheat Noodles with Vegetables

Ingredients

- 1/3 lb buckwheat (soba) noodles
- 2 cups frozen, shelled edamame beans
- 1 teaspoon olive oil
- 1 large carrot, julienned
- 1 red bell pepper, julienned
- 1 head of broccoli, broken into small florets, stems diced
- 3 Lebanese cucumbers, cut into half-moons
- 2 green onions, chopped
- 3 tablespoons tbsp. fresh cilantro, chopped

Vinaigrette

- 2 tablespoons olive oil
- 1 tablespoon apple cider vinegar
- 1 tablespoon maple syrup (preferably amber syrup for its rich flavour)

- 1 tablespoon fresh ginger, grated
- 1 teaspoon toasted sesame oil
- 1/2 teaspoon hot chili paste (like sambal oelek)

Directions

- In a saucepan, bring water to a boil over high heat and cook noodles according to package directions.
- About 4 minutes before the end of cooking, add the edamame beans. Drain and add the oil (to prevent the noodles from sticking together). Allow to cool.
- In a large bowl, combine the noodles, beans, carrot, pepper, broccoli, cucumbers, green onions, and cilantro.
- Put all the vinaigrette ingredients into a small

container with a lid. Seal
tightly and shake well.

- Pour vinaigrette over the salad
and toss well.

Cilantro Lime Cauliflower Rice

Total Time: 20 minutes

Serves: 6

Ingredients

- 1 tablespoon olive oil
- 1/2 cup white onion, chopped
- 1 large clove garlic (about 1 teaspoon)
- 1 green jalapeño deseeded & chopped (optional)
- 3 cups riced cauliflower (about 1 medium head)
- 2 tablespoons vegetable stock
- 1/2 teaspoon salt (or as needed)
- zest from 1/2 lime
- 1/2 cup fresh cilantro, chopped and divided

- 1 tablespoon lime juice

Directions

- Heat up the olive oil in a large skillet. When the oil is hot add the onions and sauté for 4-5 minutes on a medium heat or until they become soft and translucent.
- Add the garlic jalapeño and cook for a minute until the garlic becomes fragrant. Stir the whole time.
- Add the cauliflower to the skillet. Stir to mix everything together well.
- Stir in the vegetable stock, about half the cilantro salt and zest. Turn the heat up to high and cook for another minute. The high heat will draw out excess moisture in the cauliflower so it doesn't get too mushy.

- Lower the heat again and add the lime juice. Mix in to the rice well.
- Taste and season with more salt as needed. Stir in the remaining cilantro. Serve warm and enjoy!

Chicken and Rice Salad

Total Time: 15 minutes

Serves: 4

Ingredients

- 3 tablespoons olive oil
- 2 tablespoons fresh lemon juice
- 1 teaspoon finely grated lemon zest
- Kosher salt and freshly ground pepper (to taste)
- 2 cups diced cooked chicken
- 2 cups cooked rice (any kind)
- 1 cup diced celery
- 1 cup diced zucchini
- ½ cup chopped red onion

- ½ cup chopped parsley

Directions

- In a large bowl, combine the olive oil, lemon juice, lemon zest, salt, and pepper.
- Add the cooked chicken, rice, celery, zucchini, onion, and parsley. Toss to combine well. Serve at room temperature.

Honey-Ginger Sweet Potatoes

Total Time: 40 minutes

Serves: 6

Ingredients

- 1/2 cup Sue Bee Honey
- 3 pounds sweet potatoes, peeled and cubed
- 3 Tablespoons grated fresh ginger
- 2 Tablespoons walnut oil
- 1 teaspoon ground cardamom

- 1/2 teaspoon ground black pepper

Directions

- Preheat oven to 400 F.
- In a large bowl, toss together honey, sweet potatoes, ginger, walnut oil, cardamom and pepper.
- Transfer to a large cast-iron frying pan.
- Bake for 20 minutes in the preheated oven.
- Stir the potatoes to expose the pieces from the bottom of the pan.
- Bake for another 20 minutes or until the sweet potatoes are tender and caramelized on the outside.

Total Time: **22 minutes**

Serves: 4

Ingredients

- 1 1/2 tbsp olive oil (or butter)
- 2 garlic cloves, finely chopped
- 1/2 brown onion, finely chopped
- 1 1/4 tsp dried basil
- 1 cup (180g) long grain white rice, uncooked (Note 1)
- 1 3/4 cups (435 ml) chicken broth, full salt (or Veg broth)
- 2 1/2 tbsp tomato paste
- 3/4 tsp paprika, sweet or normal (not smoked)
- 1 tsp sugar (any)
- 1 sprig of basil with leaves
- 1/3 cup finely chopped basil

Directions

- Heat oil in a large saucepan over medium heat. Add garlic and onion, cook until translucent, 2 - 3 minutes. Add basil and cook for 20 seconds - don't let it burn.

- Add remaining ingredients except basil. Mix until tomato paste is dissolved.

- Crush basil sprig in hand, drop on surface then push in (leave on surface, don't stir).

- Cover and bring to simmer, then immediately turn down heat to medium low (or low if stove is strong) and cook for 15 minutes or until liquid is fully absorbed - tilt saucepan to check.

- Remove from heat and set aside, covered, for 10 minutes.

- Remove basil sprig. Fluff with fork, taste for salt. Then leave to stand for another 5 minutes, uncovered. Stir through fresh basil. Serve immediately.

Garlic Lemon Tuna Pasta

Ingredients

- 8 ounces spaghetti or other pasta
- 2 tablespoons olive oil
- 3 garlic cloves minced
- 2 pouches 2.6 ounces tuna in olive oil
- 1 tablespoon lemon juice plus zest
- Salt and pepper
- 2 tablespoons capers
- 2 tablespoons fresh parsley chopped divided
- Grated parmesan for serving

Directions

- Bring a large pot of salted water to a boil. Add the pasta and cook according to package instructions until al dente. Reserve ½ cup pasta cooking water, then drain the pasta. Return to the pot to keep warm.

- In the wide pan, heat the olive oil at medium heat. Then add the garlic and cook until fragrant, about 30 seconds. Stir in the tuna, lemon juice and zest, salt and pepper, and heat through for 1 minute.

- Add the pasta, capers and 1 tablespoon chopped parsley, and continue to stir until the spaghetti is well coated. Add as much of the reserved pasta water as needed to thin out the sauce.

One Pan Crispy Walnut Herb Chicken and Vegetables

Total Time: 35 minutes

Serves: 4

Ingredients

- 4 (6-ounce) chicken breast cutlets
- 1/4 cup whole milk
- 2 tablespoons Dijon mustard
- 1/3 cup California walnuts
- 1/3 cup panko bread crumbs
- 1 tablespoon dried parsley
- 2 teaspoons dried basil
- 2 tablespoons grated Parmesan cheese
- 1 teaspoon dried rosemary
- 1/4 teaspoon, plus 1/8 teaspoon kosher salt, divided
- 1/4 teaspoon, plus 1/8 teaspoon freshly ground black pepper, divided

- 1 cup baby potatoes, quartered (4 ounces)
- 1 cup carrots, sliced in half lengthwise
- 1 cup broccoli pieces
- 1 red bell pepper, cut into small chunks
- 1 yellow bell pepper, cut into small chunks
- 2 tablespoons olive oil

Directions

- Preheat oven to 400°F. Line a large baking sheet with aluminum foil and spray with cooking spray. Set aside.
- Pound the chicken breasts so that they are about ½-inch thick. In a shallow dish, combine milk and Dijon mustard stirring with a whisk. Add the chicken to the milk turning to coat. Set aside.

- Pulse walnuts in a food processor until they resemble fine crumbs.
- In another shallow dish, combine finely chopped walnuts with the panko bread crumbs, parsley, basil, Parmesan cheese, rosemary and 1/4 teaspoon salt and 1/4 teaspoon black pepper.
- Remove chicken from milk mixture and dredge in crumb mixture. Lay the chicken on top of the aluminum foil lined baking sheet.
- Arrange potatoes, carrots, broccoli and bell peppers around the chicken and sprinkle with 1/8 teaspoon kosher salt and 1/8 teaspoon black pepper. Drizzle olive oil over the chicken and vegetables.
- Bake for 15 minutes, then remove from oven and flip chicken and

stir veggies. Bake for an additional 15 minutes or until chicken is no longer pink. Serve immediately.

Salmon with crunchy slaw and macadamias

Ingredients

- 1 1/2 tbsp olive oil, divided
- 4 x 180g Coles Deli Fresh Salmon Skin-On, patted dry
- 1 lime, zest finely grated, juiced
- 2 tsp honey
- 200g wombok (Chinese cabbage), thinly sliced (about 4 cups)
- 200g seedless white grapes, halved
- 1 yellow capsicum, seeded, very thinly sliced

- 2 spring onions, very thinly sliced
- 1/2 cup fresh coriander leaves
- 1/2 cup fresh mint leaves
- 1/2 cup (70g) macadamias, toasted, coarsely chopped
- Lime wedges, to serve

Directions

- In a large heavy non-stick frying pan over medium heat, heat 1/2 tablespoon of the oil and then add the salmon, skin-side down. Cook for 5 mins or until the salmon skin is crisp. Turn the salmon over and cook for 2-3 mins or until salmon is mostly opaque with a rosy centre.
- Meanwhile, in a large bowl, whisk lime zest, 2 tablespoons of the lime juice, honey, remaining 1 tablespoon oil and

1/4 teaspoon salt. Add the wombok, grapes, capsicum, spring onions, coriander and mint and toss to combine. Season with salt and pepper.

- Divide the slaw among 4 plates and top with the salmon. Sprinkle the macadamias over the slaw and serve with lime wedges.

Jerk Chicken, Tomato Salsa & Sweetcorn Buckwheat

Total Time: 25 minutes

Serves: 1

Ingredients

- 80g buckwheat
- 2 free-range British chicken breasts
- 1 green chilli
- 1 handful of fresh coriander
- 1 lime
- 1 red onion (use half)

- 1 red pepper
- 1 tbsp jerk seasoning
- 140g sweetcorn
- 110g seasonal tomatoes

Directions

- Heat a large saucepan on medium heat, add the buckwheat and toast for 1 min. Fill the pan with salted hot water. Bring to a boil and cook for 10-12 mins, until cooked, then drain. Return to the pan and set aside.
- To butterfly the chicken, carefully slice through one side of each breast from the thickest part to the thinnest, careful not to cut right through to the end. Open out the chicken breasts to resemble a butterfly. Place in a bowl with 1 tbsp oil, the jerk seasoning and a pinch of sea salt. Mix to coat.

- Heat a griddle or frying pan on medium-high heat. Add the chicken and cook for 5-10 mins, per side, until cooked through.
- Make the salsa. Finely dice half the onion and tomatoes. Finely chop the chilli (remove the seeds for less heat). Place everything in a bowl and mix with the juice from half the lime, a pinch of sea salt and black pepper.
- Roughly dice the pepper. Roughly chop the coriander. Drain the sweetcorn. Add everything to the saucepan with the cooked buckwheat. Season with sea salt and black pepper and mix.
- Serve the veggie buckwheat on plates topped with the chicken and salsa. Squeeze over the remaining lime juice.

Total Time: 20 minutes

Serves: 6

Ingredients

- 2 pounds 12-15 or 16-20 count raw shrimp, peeled and deveined
- 2-3 tablespoons olive oil
- 3 cloves garlic minced
- 3 lemons sliced
- ½ teaspoon kosher salt
- ½ teaspoon freshly ground black pepper

Directions

- Preheat the oven to 400 degrees F.
- In a large bowl, toss the shrimp, garlic and ⅔ of the lemon slices with 2 tablespoons of the olive oil and the salt & pepper.

- Arrange the shrimp in 1 layer on a rimmed sheet pan, ensuring that the lemon slices are spread evenly throughout. Roast for 8 to 10 minutes, just until pink and firm and cooked through.
- Serve alone or over gluten free pasta or rice.

CONCLUSION

From deciphering the fundamentals of cirrhosis-friendly nutrition to creating a kitchen that echoes with support, our quest has become a gastronomic tapestry. These culinary sections provide recipes for delectable soups, stews, appetizers, main courses, side dishes, and desserts. Nutrient density, easy digestion, and a friendly liver are the three guiding concepts that are carefully considered when preparing each meal. The tale builds to a climax with the introduction of important supplements and vitamin-rich foods, highlighting a comprehensive approach to cirrhosis management. Recognizing the individualized nature of dietary needs, I beg you to engage in a symphony of communication and vigilance with healthcare specialists, resulting in a personalized concerto adapted to your specific needs.

As you embark on your culinary journey, consider this work to be more than just a collection of recipes. It encourages you to make wise and health-conscious decisions, emphasizing that by establishing a diet of balance and nourishment, you may improve your well-being in the face of cirrhosis's challenges.

In summary, this strives to be your wise companion, an ally who provides not just gourmet inspiration but also a wellspring of insight. May it direct your gastronomic journey to a haven of optimal liver health and profound well-being.